ALLEN SMITH

8 Weeks to 30 Consecutive Pull-Ups

Build Your Upper Body Working Your Upper Back, Shoulders, and Biceps | at Home Workouts | No Gym Required |

First published by Nelaco Press 2021

The exercises provided by the author (and the publisher) are for educational and entertainment purposes only and are not to be interpreted as a recommendation for a specific course of action. Exercise is not without its risks, and this or any other exercise program may result in injury. They include but are not limited to: risk of injury, aggravation of a pre-existing condition, or adverse effect of over-exertion such as muscle strain, abnormal blood pressure, fainting, disorders of heartbeat, and very rare instances of heart attack.

To reduce the risk of injury, before beginning this or any exercise program, please consult a healthcare provider for appropriate exercise prescription and safety precautions. The exercises instructions and advice presented are in no way intended as a substitute for medical consultation. The author (and the publisher) disclaims any liability from and in connection with this program. As with any exercise program, if at any point during your workout you begin to feel faint, dizzy, or have physical discomfort, you should stop immediately and consult a physician.

First edition

ISBN: 978-1-952381-12-6

This book was professionally typeset on Reedsy.
Find out more at reedsy.com

Contents

Before You Begin

Hey reader, thanks for grabbing a copy of the book.

If you are looking to pair this workout program with a complimentary guide to shed weight and boost your growth hormones to build more muscle faster, then I've got you covered.

Seems crazy to do both at the same time, but you can.

Better still, it is stupid easy.

Oh, and it is free. You can do this method anytime you want, anywhere for the rest of your life.

I usually sell this information, but I want you to have it.

You can get a copy from your cell phone from a simple text.

Seriously, get your phone out and text BOOST to (678) 506-7543.

Cheers!

Introduction - How to Use This Book

I will just come out and say it, pull-ups are, hands down, one of the greatest, if not the greatest, bodyweight exercise.

It is the equalizer of all exercises.

Sure, it looks cool to be able to bench press over 200 lbs but if you cannot pull off 10 pull-ups then I am not impressed.

When people ask me, what is the fastest way to get stronger? I always tell them pull-ups.

What people do not realize is pull-ups can be your "secret sauce" to upping your gains and staying out of plateaus across the board.

And sadly, you would be hard-pressed to find a lot of people even in a gym who can do even 10 consecutive pull-ups.

But we are not here to shoot for a mere 10. We are going straight for 30. A feat hardly anyone can do.

And that's exactly what we are going to tackle here in this 8-week program.

Sure, you could do pull-ups on your own, try and knock out as many as possible every day and work your way to 30 but you are either going to fall short or give up before you even get there.

What you need is strategically designed workouts for your current fitness level that challenge you just enough without killing you. Each workout will push you for the proper progression to make steady gains along the way. This program is structured to take all the guesswork out of your journey to 30 consecutive pull-ups.

And these workouts can literally be completed anywhere as long as you have a sturdy bar to complete your reps.

You will begin your journey with an initial assessment to determine your current max pull-up count. From there, you will be guided to your first workout to get started.

Once you complete the program, you will have earned the right to attempt the 30 pull-ups in a row. Some people knock it out in the first attempt. Others need a few more weeks of training.

What I can promise you is if you put in the work, you will see the results.

Up next is the initial assessment. Get after it, champ.

Initial Pull-up Assessment

This is the first step into your incredible journey to doing 30 consecutive pull-ups. It will be hard but manageable as you embark on something that very few people on the face of the earth have ever accomplished.

We are going to start out with a pull-up assessment to determine where you should start in the program.

As you can imagine, you will need a pull-up bar to complete your assessment so go ahead and find one handy to get started.

Make sure you are doing full pull-ups going all the way through the motion palms facing away from you. Starting at the bottom with arms straight and shoulders engaged, pull up to the bar so your chin goes over the bar. Then descend back down in a controlled manner to the start position.

Alright, you should be near a pull-up bar. Go ahead and complete as many pull-ups as you can without stopping.

Once you are done, write down the number of fully completed pull-ups below and head to the post-assessment results section.

Note: If this is the first assessment, you will write your assessment number in the '1ˢᵗ assessment' row. When you come back to do another assessment, you write in your completed number of reps in the respective row depending on how many assessments you have completed.

_____ reps: 1st assessment

_____ reps: 2nd assessment

_____ reps: 3rd assessment

_____ reps: 4th assessment

_____ reps: 5th assessment

_____ reps: 6th assessment

_____ reps: 7th assessment

_____ reps: 8th assessment

_____ reps: 9th assessment

_____ reps: 10th assessment

_____ reps: 11th assessment

_____ reps: 12th assessment

_____ reps: 13th assessment

_____ reps: 14th assessment

_____ reps: 15th assessment

_____ reps: 16th assessment

_____ reps: 17th assessment

_____ reps: 18th assessment

_____ reps: 19th assessment

_____ reps: 20th assessment

Post-Assessment Results

So...how did you do?

Were you surprised with how many you did or were you underwhelmed and disappointed that you did not do so hot?

Do not beat yourself up. This is simply a baseline for you to start from.

With your score in mind, you are now going to be directed to your workout grouping based on your score.

Do not get too caught up in the name of each group of workouts, these are just fun names to identify which group you are currently in. If you do not like your current group name, do not worry, stick with the program long enough and you will be out of that group in no time and into another group whose name you probably will not like either.

Before I go into informing you of your baseline workout, I recommend leaving a day between now and hitting your first workout to recover from your assessment. However, you do not have to if you are feeling gung-ho and want to go ahead and knock out your first workout.

- If you did 2 or less, you will start in the Foundation Group to build up your strength
- If you did 3, you will start in the Novice Group

- If you did between 4 and 5, you will start in the Newb Group
- If you did between 6 and 7, you will start in the Greenhorn Group
- If you did between 8 and 9, you will start in the Cub Group
- If you did between 10 and 11, you will start in the Rookie Group
- If you did between 12 and 13, you will start in the Pleb Group
- If you did between 14 and 15, you will start in the Gorilla Group
- If you did between 16 and 17, you will start in the Viking Group
- If you did between 18 and 19, you will start in the Elite Group
- If you did between 20 and 21, you will start in the Commando Group
- If you did between 22 and 23, you will start in the Veteran Group
- If you did greater than 24, you will start in the Nuclear Group

Now that you know your group, you know where you will begin for your next workout.

In your group, you will start with workout 1 followed by workout 2 and 3.

For example, let's say you completed 6 reps, and you were going to workout Monday, Wednesday, and Friday. That would put you in the greenhorn group with workout 1 on Monday, Workout 2 on Wednesday, and workout 3 on Friday.

The following week, you'd start with greenhorn group workout 4 followed by 5 and 6.

Simple enough.

Also, some of your workouts will involve what I call fundamental pull-ups.

Fundamental pull-ups involve a very slow descend and a normal ascend during the pull-up exercise. These work the full range of muscles throughout the entire pull-up. Traditional pull-ups only provide significant tensions during the pull. These pull-ups make you work during the descent and the pull. You will have either 5 or 10 second descends during your workouts.

For example, if you have a set of 3 fundamental pull-ups with 5 seconds descends, you will start in the up, ready position and lower yourself slowly over a 5 second period to the bottom of the exercise. You will then pull back up to the starting position like a normal pull-up. As soon as you get to the top of the exercise with your chin over the bar, you will begin gradually lowering yourself back down over another 5 second period for the second rep followed by the third.

These fundamental pull-ups force you to work out any weak areas. Most people perform pull-ups too fast using momentum to get their chin above the bar. This causes some muscles to get more attention than others. Oftentimes people are strong enough to do more pull-ups, but their forearms are so weak they cannot stay on the bar long enough to do it. We are going to use fundamental pull-ups to make sure that does not happen.

They do not sound bad, but boy do they start to burn quick.

Great job on your assessment and get ready for your first workout.

Workout Completion Checklist

Check off your workouts as you complete them:

_____Foundation Group Workout 1

_____Foundation Group Workout 2

_____Foundation Group Workout 3

_____Foundation Group Workout 4

_____Foundation Group Workout 5

_____Foundation Group Workout 6

_____Novice Group Workout 1

_____Novice Group Workout 2

_____Novice Group Workout 3

_____Novice Group Workout 4

_____Novice Group Workout 5

_____Novice Group Workout 6

_____Newb Group Workout 1

_____Newb Group Workout 2

_____Newb Group Workout 3

_____Newb Group Workout 4

_____Newb Group Workout 5

_____Newb Group Workout 6

_____Greenhorn Group Workout 1

_____Greenhorn Group Workout 2

_____Greenhorn Group Workout 3

_____Greenhorn Group Workout 4

_____Greenhorn Group Workout 5

_____Greenhorn Group Workout 6
_____Cub Group Workout 1
_____Cub Group Workout 2
_____Cub Group Workout 3
_____Cub Group Workout 4
_____Cub Group Workout 5
_____Cub Group Workout 6
_____Rookie Group Workout 1
_____Rookie Group Workout 2
_____Rookie Group Workout 3
_____Rookie Group Workout 4
_____Rookie Group Workout 5
_____Rookie Group Workout 6
_____Pleb Group Workout 1
_____Pleb Group Workout 2
_____Pleb Group Workout 3
_____Pleb Group Workout 4
_____Pleb Group Workout 5
_____Pleb Group Workout 6
_____Gorilla Group Workout 1
_____Gorilla Group Workout 2
_____Gorilla Group Workout 3
_____Gorilla Group Workout 4
_____Gorilla Group Workout 5
_____Gorilla Group Workout 6
_____Viking Group Workout 1
_____Viking Group Workout 2
_____Viking Group Workout 3
_____Viking Group Workout 4
_____Viking Group Workout 5
_____Viking Group Workout 6
_____Elite Group Workout 1
_____Elite Group Workout 2

_____Elite Group Workout 3

_____Elite Group Workout 4

_____Elite Group Workout 5

_____Elite Group Workout 6

_____Commando Group Workout 1

_____Commando Group Workout 2

_____Commando Group Workout 3

_____Commando Group Workout 4

_____Commando Group Workout 5

_____Commando Group Workout 6

_____Veteran Group Workout 1

_____Veteran Group Workout 2

_____Veteran Group Workout 3

_____Veteran Group Workout 4

_____Veteran Group Workout 5

_____Veteran Group Workout 6

_____Nuclear Group Workout 1

_____Nuclear Group Workout 2

_____Nuclear Group Workout 3

_____Nuclear Group Workout 4

_____Nuclear Group Workout 5

_____Nuclear Group Workout 6

_____Attempting 30 Consecutive Pull-ups

_____Completed 30 Consecutive Pull-ups: _____ reps.

Pre & Post Program Measurements

The following measurements are 100% optional and are not required to start or finish the program. I know some people will be curious to know other areas that are positively affected by achieving 30 consecutive pull-ups.

Starting weight: _____

Starting body row rep max: _____

Starting standing row max: _____

Starting cable pull down max: _____

Starting bicep measurement: _____

Ending weight: _____

Ending body row rep max: _____

Ending standing row max: _____

Ending cable pull down max: _____

Ending bicep measurement: _____

Foundation Group Workouts

Foundation Group Workout 1

Welcome to the Foundation Group Workout 1.

For this workout, you have 5 sets with 60 seconds of rest between each set consisting of negative pull-ups.

Negative pull-ups simply focus on the descend with no ascending pull back to the starting position. Instead of starting at the bottom of the position and pulling yourself up, you are going to jump up or stand on something so you can start at the top positive and slowly lower yourself down over a period of 3 to 10 seconds. As soon as you complete your descent, you can stop and rest.

Note: You may need something to step up on to start at the top positive if you are unable to jump up to the top position. Just make sure that whatever you stand on, just like whatever you use as pull-up bar, is sturdy.

Remember to focus on proper form throughout your sets and always start in the up, ready position.

Sets:

1. 1 negative pull-up with a 5 second descend.
2. 1 negative pull-up with a 5 second descend.
3. 1 negative pull-up with a 5 second descend.

4. 1 negative pull-up with a 5 second descend.
5. 1 negative pull-up with a 5 second descend.

If you completed this workout, head to Foundation Group Workout 2 for your next session. If not, stick with this one until you complete it.

Foundation Group Workout 2

Welcome to the Foundation Group Workout 2.

For this workout, you have 5 sets with 60 seconds of rest between each set consisting of negative pull-ups.

Rest for 1 minute between each set.

Remember to focus on proper form throughout your sets and always start on the up, ready position.

Sets:

1. 1 negative pull-up with a 7 second descend.
2. 1 negative pull-up with a 7 second descend.
3. 1 negative pull-up with a 7 second descend.
4. 1 negative pull-up with a 5 second descend.
5. 1 negative pull-up with a 5 second descend.

If you completed this workout, head to Foundation Group Workout 3 for your next session. If not, stick with this one until you complete it.

Foundation Group Workout 3

Welcome to the Foundation Group Workout 3.

For this workout, you have 5 sets with 60 seconds of rest between each set consisting of fundamental and negative pull-ups.

As I mentioned before, fundamental pull-ups involve a very slow descend. and a normal ascend during the pull-up exercise. These work the full range of muscles throughout the entire pull-ups to help build up your strength.

Rest for 1 minute between each set.

Remember to focus on proper form throughout your sets and always start on the up, ready position.

Sets:

1. 1 fundamental pull-up with a 5 second descend.
2. 1 fundamental pull-up with a 5 second descend.
3. 1 negative pull-up with a 5 second descend.
4. 1 negative pull-up with a 5 second descend.
5. 1 negative pull-up with a 5 second descend.

If you completed this workout, head to Foundation Group Workout 4 for your next session. If not, stick with this one until you complete it.

Foundation Group Workout 4

Welcome to the Foundation Group Workout 4.

For this workout, you have 5 sets with 60 seconds of rest between each set consisting of negative pull-ups.

Rest for 1 minute between each set.

Remember to focus on proper form throughout your sets and always start on the up, ready position.

Sets:

1. 1 negative pull-up with a 10 second descend.
2. 1 negative pull-up with a 10 second descend.
3. 1 negative pull-up with a 7 second descend.
4. 1 negative pull-up with a 7 second descend.
5. 1 negative pull-up with a 7 second descend.

If you completed this workout, head to Foundation Group Workout 5 for your next session. If not, stick with this one until you complete it.

Foundation Group Workout 5

Welcome to the Foundation Group Workout 5.

For this workout, you have 5 sets with 60 seconds of rest between each set consisting of fundamental and negative pull-ups.

Rest for 1 minute between each set.

Remember to focus on proper form throughout your sets and always start on the up, ready position.

Sets:

1. 1 fundamental pull-up with a 5 second descend.
2. 1 fundamental pull-up with a 5 second descend.
3. 1 fundamental pull-up with a 5 second descend.
4. 1 negative pull-up with a 5 second descend.
5. 1 negative pull-up with a 5 second descend.

If you completed this workout, head to Foundation Group Workout 6 for your next session. If not, stick with this one until you complete it.

Foundation Group Workout 6

Welcome to the Foundation Group Workout 6.

For this workout, you have 5 sets with 60 seconds of rest between each set consisting of fundamental and negative pull-ups.

Remember to focus on proper form throughout your sets and always start on the up, ready position.

Sets:

1. 1 fundamental pull-up with a 5 second descend.
2. 1 fundamental pull-up with a 5 second descend.
3. 1 fundamental pull-up with a 5 second descend.
4. 1 negative pull-up with a 7 second descend.
5. 1 negative pull-up with a 7 second descend.

Since this is the end of a two-week period, it is time to redo your pull-up assessment to check your progress. Rest a day and give the assessment a go to see which Group you will be in next.

Novice Group Workouts

Novice Group Workout 1

Welcome to the Novice Group Workout 1.

For this workout, you have 6 sets with 60 seconds of rest between each set.

Remember to focus on proper form throughout your sets.

Sets:

1. 1 pull-up
2. 1 pull-up
3. 1 pull-up
4. 1 pull-up
5. 1 pull-up
6. 1 fundamental pull-up with a 5 second descend.

If you completed this workout, head to Novice Group Workout 2 for your next session. If not, stick with this one until you complete it.

Glasses of water drank today: 1-2-3-4-5-6-7-8-9-10

Hours of sleep last night: 1-2-3-4-5-6-7-8-9-10

Diet: junk food————semi-healthy————healthy

Novice Group Workout 2

Welcome to the Novice Group Workout 2.

For this workout, you have 6 sets with 60 seconds of rest between each set.

Remember to focus on proper form throughout your sets.

Sets:

1. 1 pull-up
2. 2 pull-ups
3. 1 pull-up
4. 1 pull-up
5. 1 pull-up
6. 1 fundamental pull-up with a 5 second descend.

If you completed this workout, head to Novice Group Workout 3 for your next session. If not, stick with this one until you complete it.

Glasses of water drank today: 1-2-3-4-5-6-7-8-9-10

Hours of sleep last night: 1-2-3-4-5-6-7-8-9-10

Diet: junk food—————semi-healthy—————healthy

Novice Group Workout 3

Welcome to the Novice Group Workout 3.

For this workout, you have 6 sets with 90 seconds of rest between each set.

Remember to focus on proper form throughout your sets.

Sets:

1. 1 pull-up
2. 2 pull-ups
3. 2 pull-ups
4. 1 pull-up
5. 1 pull-up
6. Max out: perform as many pull-ups as you can.

Max reps: _____

If you completed this workout, head to Novice Group Workout 4 for your next session. If not, stick with this one until you complete it.

Glasses of water drank today: 1-2-3-4-5-6-7-8-9-10

Hours of sleep last night: 1-2-3-4-5-6-7-8-9-10

Diet: junk food—————semi-healthy—————healthy

Novice Group Workout 4

Welcome to the Novice Group Workout 4.

For this workout, you have 6 sets with 60 seconds of rest between each set.

Remember to focus on proper form throughout your sets.

Sets:

1. 1 pull-up
2. 2 pull-ups
3. 2 pull-ups
4. 2 pull-ups
5. 1 pull-up
6. 1 fundamental pull-up with a 5 second descend.

If you completed this workout, head to Novice Group Workout 5 for your next session. If not, stick with this one until you complete it.

Glasses of water drank today: 1-2-3-4-5-6-7-8-9-10

Hours of sleep last night: 1-2-3-4-5-6-7-8-9-10

Diet: junk food————semi-healthy————healthy

Novice Group Workout 5

Welcome to the Novice Group Workout 5.

For this workout, you have 6 sets with 60 seconds of rest between each set.

Remember to focus on proper form throughout your sets.

Sets:

1. 2 pull-ups
2. 2 pull-ups
3. 2 pull-ups
4. 2 pull-ups
5. 2 pull-ups
6. 1 fundamental pull-up with a 5 second descend.

If you completed this workout, head to Novice Group Workout 6 for your next session. If not, stick with this one until you complete it.

Glasses of water drank today: 1-2-3-4-5-6-7-8-9-10

Hours of sleep last night: 1-2-3-4-5-6-7-8-9-10

Diet: junk food————semi-healthy————healthy

Novice Group Workout 6

Welcome to the Novice Group Workout 6.

For this workout, you have 6 sets with 90 seconds of rest between each set.

Remember to focus on proper form throughout your sets.

Sets:

1. 2 pull-ups
2. 3 pull-ups
3. 2 pull-ups
4. 2 pull-ups
5. 2 pull-ups
6. Max out: perform as many pull-ups as you can.

Max reps: _____

Since this is the end of a two-week period, it is time to redo your pull-up assessment to check your progress if you fully completed this workout.

Rest a day and give the assessment a go to see which Group you will be in next.

Glasses of water drank today: 1-2-3-4-5-6-7-8-9-10

Hours of sleep last night: 1-2-3-4-5-6-7-8-9-10

Diet: junk food—————semi-healthy—————healthy

Newb Group Workouts

Newb Group Workout 1

Welcome to the Newb Group Workout 1.

For this workout, you have 6 sets with 60 seconds of rest between each set.

Remember to focus on proper form throughout your sets.

Sets:

1. 2 pull-ups
2. 2 pull-ups
3. 2 pull-ups
4. 2 pull-ups
5. 2 pull-ups
6. 1 fundamental pull-up with a 5 second descend.

If you completed this workout, head to Newb Group Workout 2 for your next session. If not, stick with this one until you complete it.

Glasses of water drank today: 1-2-3-4-5-6-7-8-9-10

Hours of sleep last night: 1-2-3-4-5-6-7-8-9-10

Diet: junk food—————semi-healthy—————healthy

Newb Group Workout 2

Welcome to the Newb Group Workout 2.

For this workout, you have 6 sets with 60 seconds of rest between each set.

Remember to focus on proper form throughout your sets.

Sets:

1. 2 pull-ups
2. 3 pull-ups
3. 2 pull-ups
4. 2 pull-ups
5. 2 pull-ups
6. 1 fundamental pull-up with a 5 second descend.

If you completed this workout, head to Newb Group Workout 3 for your next session. If not, stick with this one until you complete it.

Glasses of water drank today: 1-2-3-4-5-6-7-8-9-10

Hours of sleep last night: 1-2-3-4-5-6-7-8-9-10

Diet: junk food————semi-healthy————healthy

Newb Group Workout 3

Welcome to the Newb Group Workout 3.

For this workout, you have 6 sets with 90 seconds of rest between each set.

Remember to focus on proper form throughout your sets.

Sets:

1. 2 pull-ups
2. 3 pull-ups
3. 3 pull-ups
4. 2 pull-ups
5. 2 pull-ups
6. Max out: perform as many pull-ups as you can.

Max reps: _____

If you completed this workout, head to Newb Group Workout 4 for your next session. If not, stick with this one until you complete it.

Glasses of water drank today: 1-2-3-4-5-6-7-8-9-10

Hours of sleep last night: 1-2-3-4-5-6-7-8-9-10

Diet: junk food————semi-healthy————healthy

Newb Group Workout 4

Welcome to the Newb Group Workout 4.

For this workout, you have 6 sets with 60 seconds of rest between each set.

Remember to focus on proper form throughout your sets.

Sets:

1. 3 pull-ups
2. 3 pull-ups
3. 3 pull-ups
4. 3 pull-ups
5. 3 pull-ups
6. 1 fundamental pull-up with a 5 second descend.

If you completed this workout, head to Newb Group Workout 5 for your next session. If not, stick with this one until you complete it.

Glasses of water drank today: 1-2-3-4-5-6-7-8-9-10

Hours of sleep last night: 1-2-3-4-5-6-7-8-9-10

Diet: junk food—————semi-healthy—————healthy

Newb Group Workout 5

Welcome to the Newb Group Workout 5.

For this workout, you have 6 sets with 60 seconds of rest between each set.

Remember to focus on proper form throughout your sets.

Sets:

1. 3 pull-ups
2. 4 pull-ups
3. 3 pull-ups
4. 3 pull-ups
5. 3 pull-ups
6. 1 fundamental pull-up with a 5 second descend.

If you completed this workout, head to Newb Group Workout 6 for your next session. If not, stick with this one until you complete it.

Glasses of water drank today: 1-2-3-4-5-6-7-8-9-10

Hours of sleep last night: 1-2-3-4-5-6-7-8-9-10

Diet: junk food————semi-healthy————healthy

Newb Group Workout 6

Welcome to the Newb Group Workout 6.

For this workout, you have 6 sets with 90 seconds of rest between each set.

Remember to focus on proper form throughout your sets.

Sets:

1. 3 pull-ups
2. 4 pull-ups
3. 4 pull-ups
4. 3 pull-ups
5. 3 pull-ups
6. Max out: perform as many pull-ups as you can.

Max reps: _____

Since this is the end of a two-week period, it is time to redo your pull-up assessment to check your progress if you fully completed this workout.

Rest a day and give the assessment a go to see which Group you will be in next.

Glasses of water drank today: 1-2-3-4-5-6-7-8-9-10

Hours of sleep last night: 1-2-3-4-5-6-7-8-9-10

Diet: junk food————semi-healthy————healthy

Greenhorn Group Workouts

Greenhorn Group Workout 1

Welcome to the Greenhorn Group Workout 1.

For this workout, you have 6 sets with 60 seconds of rest between each set.

Remember to focus on proper form throughout your sets.

Sets:

1. 3 pull-ups
2. 3 pull-ups
3. 3 pull-ups
4. 3 pull-ups
5. 3 pull-ups
6. 1 fundamental pull-up with a 5 second descend.

If you completed this workout, head to Greenhorn Group Workout 2 for your next session. If not, stick with this one until you complete it.

Glasses of water drank today: 1-2-3-4-5-6-7-8-9-10

Hours of sleep last night: 1-2-3-4-5-6-7-8-9-10

Diet: junk food————semi-healthy————healthy

Greenhorn Group Workout 2

Welcome to the Greenhorn Group Workout 2.

For this workout, you have 6 sets with 60 seconds of rest between each set.

Remember to focus on proper form throughout your sets.

Sets:

1. 3 pull-ups
2. 4 pull-ups
3. 3 pull-ups
4. 3 pull-ups
5. 3 pull-ups
6. 1 fundamental pull-up with a 5 second descend.

If you completed this workout, head to Greenhorn Group Workout 3 for your next session. If not, stick with this one until you complete it.

Glasses of water drank today: 1-2-3-4-5-6-7-8-9-10

Hours of sleep last night: 1-2-3-4-5-6-7-8-9-10

Diet: junk food————semi-healthy————healthy

Greenhorn Group Workout 3

Welcome to the Greenhorn Group Workout 3.

For this workout, you have 6 sets with 90 seconds of rest between each set.

Remember to focus on proper form throughout your sets.

Sets:

1. 3 pull-ups
2. 4 pull-ups
3. 4 pull-ups
4. 3 pull-ups
5. 3 pull-ups
6. Max out: perform as many pull-ups as you can.

Max reps: _____

If you completed this workout, head to Greenhorn Group Workout 4 for your next session. If not, stick with this one until you complete it.

Glasses of water drank today: 1-2-3-4-5-6-7-8-9-10

Hours of sleep last night: 1-2-3-4-5-6-7-8-9-10

Diet: junk food—————semi-healthy—————healthy

Greenhorn Group Workout 4

Welcome to the Greenhorn Group Workout 4.

For this workout, you have 6 sets with 60 seconds of rest between each set.

Remember to focus on proper form throughout your sets.

Sets:

1. 4 pull-ups
2. 4 pull-ups
3. 4 pull-ups
4. 4 pull-ups
5. 4 pull-ups
6. 1 fundamental pull-up with a 5 second descend.

If you completed this workout, head to Greenhorn Group Workout 5 for your next session. If not, stick with this one until you complete it.

Glasses of water drank today: 1-2-3-4-5-6-7-8-9-10

Hours of sleep last night: 1-2-3-4-5-6-7-8-9-10

Diet: junk food—————semi-healthy—————healthy

Greenhorn Group Workout 5

Welcome to the Greenhorn Group Workout 5.

For this workout, you have 6 sets with 60 seconds of rest between each set.

Remember to focus on proper form throughout your sets.

Sets:

1. 4 pull-ups
2. 5 pull-ups
3. 5 pull-ups
4. 4 pull-ups
5. 4 pull-ups
6. 1 fundamental pull-up with a 5 second descend.

If you completed this workout, head to Greenhorn Group Workout 6 for your next session. If not, stick with this one until you complete it.

Glasses of water drank today: 1-2-3-4-5-6-7-8-9-10

Hours of sleep last night: 1-2-3-4-5-6-7-8-9-10

Diet: junk food————semi-healthy————healthy

Greenhorn Group Workout 6

Welcome to the Greenhorn Group Workout 6.

For this workout, you have 6 sets with 90 seconds of rest between each set.

Remember to focus on proper form throughout your sets.

Sets:

1. 5 pull-ups
2. 5 pull-ups
3. 5 pull-ups
4. 5 pull-ups
5. 5 pull-ups
6. Max out: perform as many pull-ups as you can.

Max reps: _____

Since this is the end of a two-week period, it is time to redo your pull-up assessment to check your progress if you fully completed this workout.

Rest a day and give the assessment a go to see which Group you will be in next.

Glasses of water drank today: 1-2-3-4-5-6-7-8-9-10

Hours of sleep last night: 1-2-3-4-5-6-7-8-9-10

Diet: junk food————semi-healthy————healthy

Cub Group Workouts

Cub Group Workout 1

Welcome to the Cub Group Workout 1.

For this workout, you have 6 sets with 60 seconds of rest between each set.

Remember to focus on proper form throughout your sets.

Sets:

1. 2 pull-ups
2. 3 pull-ups
3. 3 pull-ups
4. 3 pull-ups
5. 2 pull-ups
6. 1 fundamental pull-up with a 10 second descend.

If you completed this workout, head to Cub Group Workout 2 for your next session. If not, stick with this one until you complete it.

Glasses of water drank today: 1-2-3-4-5-6-7-8-9-10

Hours of sleep last night: 1-2-3-4-5-6-7-8-9-10

Diet: junk food————semi-healthy————healthy

Cub Group Workout 2

Welcome to the Cub Group Workout 2.

For this workout, you have 6 sets with 60 seconds of rest between each set.

Remember to focus on proper form throughout your sets.

Sets:

1. 3 pull-ups
2. 3 pull-ups
3. 3 pull-ups
4. 3 pull-ups
5. 3 pull-ups
6. 1 fundamental pull-up with a 10 second descend.

If you completed this workout, head to Cub Group Workout 3 for your next session. If not, stick with this one until you complete it.

Glasses of water drank today: 1-2-3-4-5-6-7-8-9-10

Hours of sleep last night: 1-2-3-4-5-6-7-8-9-10

Diet: junk food————semi-healthy————healthy

Cub Group Workout 3

Welcome to the Cub Group Workout 3.

For this workout, you have 6 sets with 90 seconds of rest between each set.

Remember to focus on proper form throughout your sets.

Sets:

1. 3 pull-ups
2. 4 pull-ups
3. 4 pull-ups
4. 3 pull-ups
5. 3 pull-ups
6. Max out: perform as many pull-ups as you can.

Max reps: _____

If you completed this workout, head to Cub Group Workout 4 for your next session. If not, stick with this one until you complete it.

Glasses of water drank today: 1-2-3-4-5-6-7-8-9-10

Hours of sleep last night: 1-2-3-4-5-6-7-8-9-10

Diet: junk food————semi-healthy————healthy

Cub Group Workout 4

Welcome to the Cub Group Workout 4.

For this workout, you have 6 sets with 60 seconds of rest between each set.

Remember to focus on proper form throughout your sets.

Sets:

1. 4 pull-ups
2. 4 pull-ups
3. 4 pull-ups
4. 4 pull-ups
5. 4 pull-ups
6. 1 fundamental pull-up with a 10 second descend.

If you completed this workout, head to Cub Group Workout 5 for your next session. If not, stick with this one until you complete it.

Glasses of water drank today: 1-2-3-4-5-6-7-8-9-10

Hours of sleep last night: 1-2-3-4-5-6-7-8-9-10

Diet: junk food—————semi-healthy—————healthy

Cub Group Workout 5

Welcome to the Cub Group Workout 5.

For this workout, you have 6 sets with 60 seconds of rest between each set.

Remember to focus on proper form throughout your sets.

Sets:

1. 4 pull-ups
2. 5 pull-ups
3. 5 pull-ups
4. 4 pull-ups
5. 4 pull-ups
6. 1 fundamental pull-up with a 10 second descend.

If you completed this workout, head to Cub Group Workout 6 for your next session. If not, stick with this one until you complete it.

Glasses of water drank today: 1-2-3-4-5-6-7-8-9-10

Hours of sleep last night: 1-2-3-4-5-6-7-8-9-10

Diet: junk food————semi-healthy————healthy

Cub Group Workout 6

Welcome to the Cub Group Workout 6.

For this workout, you have 6 sets with 90 seconds of rest between each set.

Remember to focus on proper form throughout your sets.

Sets:

1. 5 pull-ups
2. 5 pull-ups
3. 5 pull-ups
4. 5 pull-ups
5. 5 pull-ups
6. Max out: perform as many pull-ups as you can.

Max reps: _____

Since this is the end of a two-week period, it is time to redo your pull-up assessment to check your progress if you fully completed this workout.

Rest a day and give the assessment a go to see which Group you will be in next.

Glasses of water drank today: 1-2-3-4-5-6-7-8-9-10

Hours of sleep last night: 1-2-3-4-5-6-7-8-9-10

Diet: junk food————semi-healthy————healthy

Rookie Group Workouts

Rookie Group Workout 1

Welcome to the Rookie Group Workout 1.

For this workout, you have 6 sets with 60 seconds of rest between each set.

Remember to focus on proper form throughout your sets.

Sets:

1. 4 pull-ups
2. 4 pull-ups
3. 4 pull-ups
4. 4 pull-ups
5. 4 pull-ups
6. 1 fundamental pull-up with a 10 second descend.

If you completed this workout, head to Cub Group Workout 2 for your next session. If not, stick with this one until you complete it.

Glasses of water drank today: 1-2-3-4-5-6-7-8-9-10

Hours of sleep last night: 1-2-3-4-5-6-7-8-9-10

Diet: junk food—————semi-healthy—————healthy

Rookie Group Workout 2

Welcome to the Rookie Group Workout 2.

For this workout, you have 6 sets with 60 seconds of rest between each set.

Remember to focus on proper form throughout your sets.

Sets:

1. 5 pull-ups
2. 5 pull-ups
3. 5 pull-ups
4. 5 pull-ups
5. 5 pull-ups
6. 1 fundamental pull-up with a 10 second descend.

If you completed this workout, head to Rookie Group Workout 3 for your next session. If not, stick with this one until you complete it.

Glasses of water drank today: 1-2-3-4-5-6-7-8-9-10

Hours of sleep last night: 1-2-3-4-5-6-7-8-9-10

Diet: junk food————semi-healthy————healthy

Rookie Group Workout 3

Welcome to the Rookie Group Workout 3.

For this workout, you have 6 sets with 90 seconds of rest between each set.

Remember to focus on proper form throughout your sets.

Sets:

1. 5 pull-ups
2. 6 pull-ups
3. 6 pull-ups
4. 5 pull-ups
5. 5 pull-ups
6. Max out: perform as many pull-ups as you can.

Max reps: _____

If you completed this workout, head to Rookie Group Workout 4 for your next session. If not, stick with this one until you complete it.

Glasses of water drank today: 1-2-3-4-5-6-7-8-9-10

Hours of sleep last night: 1-2-3-4-5-6-7-8-9-10

Diet: junk food—————semi-healthy—————healthy

Rookie Group Workout 4

Welcome to the Rookie Group Workout 4.

For this workout, you have 6 sets with 60 seconds of rest between each set.

Remember to focus on proper form throughout your sets.

Sets:

1. 6 pull-ups
2. 6 pull-ups
3. 6 pull-ups
4. 6 pull-ups
5. 6 pull-ups
6. 2 fundamental pull-ups with a 10 second descend.

If you completed this workout, head to Rookie Group Workout 5 for your next session. If not, stick with this one until you complete it.

Glasses of water drank today: 1-2-3-4-5-6-7-8-9-10

Hours of sleep last night: 1-2-3-4-5-6-7-8-9-10

Diet: junk food—————semi-healthy—————healthy

Rookie Group Workout 5

Welcome to the Rookie Group Workout 5.

For this workout, you have 6 sets with 60 seconds of rest between each set.

Remember to focus on proper form throughout your sets.

Sets:

1. 7 pull-ups
2. 7 pull-ups
3. 7 pull-ups
4. 7 pull-ups
5. 7 pull-ups
6. 2 fundamental pull-ups with a 10 second descend.

If you completed this workout, head to Rookie Group Workout 6 for your next session. If not, stick with this one until you complete it.

Glasses of water drank today: 1-2-3-4-5-6-7-8-9-10

Hours of sleep last night: 1-2-3-4-5-6-7-8-9-10

Diet: junk food—————semi-healthy—————healthy

Rookie Group Workout 6

Welcome to the Rookie Group Workout 6.

For this workout, you have 6 sets with 90 seconds of rest between each set.

Remember to focus on proper form throughout your sets.

Sets:

1. 7 pull-ups
2. 8 pull-ups
3. 8 pull-ups
4. 7 pull-ups
5. 7 pull-ups
6. Max out: perform as many pull-ups as you can.

Max reps: _____

Since this is the end of a two-week period, it is time to redo your pull-up assessment to check your progress if you fully completed this workout.

Rest a day and give the assessment a go to see which Group you will be in next.

Glasses of water drank today: 1-2-3-4-5-6-7-8-9-10

Hours of sleep last night: 1-2-3-4-5-6-7-8-9-10

Diet: junk food————semi-healthy————healthy

Pleb Group Workouts

Pleb Group Workout 1

Welcome to the Pleb Group Workout 1.

For this workout, you have 6 sets with 60 seconds of rest between each set.

Remember to focus on proper form throughout your sets.

Sets:

1. 5 pull-ups
2. 6 pull-ups
3. 6 pull-ups
4. 5 pull-ups
5. 5 pull-ups
6. 1 fundamental pull-up with a 10 second descend.

If you completed this workout, head to Pleb Group Workout 2 for your next session. If not, stick with this one until you complete it.

Glasses of water drank today: 1-2-3-4-5-6-7-8-9-10

Hours of sleep last night: 1-2-3-4-5-6-7-8-9-10

Diet: junk food————semi-healthy————healthy

Pleb Group Workout 2

Welcome to the Pleb Group Workout 2.

For this workout, you have 6 sets with 60 seconds of rest between each set.

Remember to focus on proper form throughout your sets.

Sets:

1. 6 pull-ups
2. 6 pull-ups
3. 6 pull-ups
4. 6 pull-ups
5. 6 pull-ups
6. 2 fundamental pull-ups with a 10 second descend.

If you completed this workout, head to Pleb Group Workout 3 for your next session. If not, stick with this one until you complete it.

Glasses of water drank today: 1-2-3-4-5-6-7-8-9-10

Hours of sleep last night: 1-2-3-4-5-6-7-8-9-10

Diet: junk food————semi-healthy————healthy

Pleb Group Workout 3

Welcome to the Pleb Group Workout 3.

For this workout, you have 6 sets with 90 seconds of rest between each set.

Remember to focus on proper form throughout your sets.

Sets:

1. 6 pull-ups
2. 7 pull-ups
3. 7 pull-ups
4. 6 pull-ups
5. 6 pull-ups
6. Max out: perform as many pull-ups as you can.

Max reps: _____

If you completed this workout, head to Pleb Group Workout 4 for your next session. If not, stick with this one until you complete it.

Glasses of water drank today: 1-2-3-4-5-6-7-8-9-10

Hours of sleep last night: 1-2-3-4-5-6-7-8-9-10

Diet: junk food————semi-healthy————healthy

Pleb Group Workout 4

Welcome to the Pleb Group Workout 4.

For this workout, you have 6 sets with 60 seconds of rest between each set.

Remember to focus on proper form throughout your sets.

Sets:

1. 7 pull-ups
2. 7 pull-ups
3. 7 pull-ups
4. 7 pull-ups
5. 7 pull-ups
6. 2 fundamental pull-ups with a 10 second descend.

If you completed this workout, head to Pleb Group Workout 5 for your next session. If not, stick with this one until you complete it.

Glasses of water drank today: 1-2-3-4-5-6-7-8-9-10

Hours of sleep last night: 1-2-3-4-5-6-7-8-9-10

Diet: junk food————semi-healthy————healthy

Pleb Group Workout 5

Welcome to the Pleb Group Workout 5.

For this workout, you have 6 sets with 60 seconds of rest between each set.

Remember to focus on proper form throughout your sets.

Sets:

1. 8 pull-ups
2. 8 pull-ups
3. 8 pull-ups
4. 8 pull-ups
5. 8 pull-ups
6. 2 fundamental pull-ups with a 10 second descend.

If you completed this workout, head to Pleb Group Workout 6 for your next session. If not, stick with this one until you complete it.

Glasses of water drank today: 1-2-3-4-5-6-7-8-9-10

Hours of sleep last night: 1-2-3-4-5-6-7-8-9-10

Diet: junk food—————semi-healthy—————healthy

Pleb Group Workout 6

Welcome to the Pleb Group Workout 6.

For this workout, you have 6 sets with 90 seconds of rest between each set.

Remember to focus on proper form throughout your sets.

Sets:

1. 9 pull-ups
2. 9 pull-ups
3. 9 pull-ups
4. 9 pull-ups
5. 9 pull-ups
6. Max out: perform as many pull-ups as you can.

Max reps: _____

Since this is the end of a two-week period, it is time to redo your pull-up assessment to check your progress if you fully completed this workout.

Rest a day and give the assessment a go to see which Group you will be in next.

Glasses of water drank today: 1-2-3-4-5-6-7-8-9-10

Hours of sleep last night: 1-2-3-4-5-6-7-8-9-10

Diet: junk food———————semi-healthy———————healthy

Gorilla Group Workouts

Gorilla Group Workout 1

Welcome to the Gorilla Group Workout 1.

For this workout, you have 6 sets with 120 seconds of rest between each set.

Remember to focus on proper form throughout your sets.

Sets:

1. 5 pull-ups
2. 6 pull-ups
3. 6 pull-ups
4. 6 pull-ups
5. 5 pull-ups
6. 1 fundamental pull-up with a 10 second descend.

If you completed this workout, head to Gorilla Group Workout 2 for your next session. If not, stick with this one until you complete it.

Glasses of water drank today: 1-2-3-4-5-6-7-8-9-10

Hours of sleep last night: 1-2-3-4-5-6-7-8-9-10

Diet: junk food————semi-healthy————healthy

Gorilla Group Workout 2

Welcome to the Gorilla Group Workout 2.

For this workout, you have 9 sets with 90 seconds of rest between each set.

Remember to focus on proper form throughout your sets.

Sets:

1. 3 pull-ups
2. 4 pull-ups
3. 4 pull-ups
4. 4 pull-ups
5. 3 pull-ups
6. 3 pull-ups
7. 3 pull-ups
8. 3 pull-ups
9. 2 fundamental pull-ups with a 10 second descend.

If you completed this workout, head to Gorilla Group Workout 3 for your next session. If not, stick with this one until you complete it.

Glasses of water drank today: 1-2-3-4-5-6-7-8-9-10

Hours of sleep last night: 1-2-3-4-5-6-7-8-9-10

Diet: junk food—————semi-healthy—————healthy

Gorilla Group Workout 3

Welcome to the Gorilla Group Workout 3.

For this workout, you have 9 sets with 90 seconds of rest between each set.

Remember to focus on proper form throughout your sets.

Sets:

1. 4 pull-ups
2. 5 pull-ups
3. 5 pull-ups
4. 5 pull-ups
5. 4 pull-ups
6. 4 pull-ups
7. 4 pull-ups
8. 4 pull-ups
9. Max out: perform as many pull-ups as you can.

Max reps: _____

If you completed this workout, head to Gorilla Group Workout 4 for your next session. If not, stick with this one until you complete it.

Glasses of water drank today: 1-2-3-4-5-6-7-8-9-10

Hours of sleep last night: 1-2-3-4-5-6-7-8-9-10

Diet: junk food————semi-healthy————healthy

Gorilla Group Workout 4

Welcome to the Gorilla Group Workout 4.

For this workout, you have 6 sets with 120 seconds of rest between each set.

Remember to focus on proper form throughout your sets.

Sets:

1. 7 pull-ups
2. 7 pull-ups
3. 7 pull-ups
4. 7 pull-ups
5. 7 pull-ups
6. 3 fundamental pull-ups with a 10 second descend.

If you completed this workout, head to Gorilla Group Workout 5 for your next session. If not, stick with this one until you complete it.

Glasses of water drank today: 1-2-3-4-5-6-7-8-9-10

Hours of sleep last night: 1-2-3-4-5-6-7-8-9-10

Diet: junk food————semi-healthy————healthy

Gorilla Group Workout 5

Welcome to the Gorilla Group Workout 5.

For this workout, you have 10 sets with 90 seconds of rest between each set.

Remember to focus on proper form throughout your sets.

Sets:

1. 4 pull-ups
2. 5 pull-ups
3. 5 pull-ups
4. 5 pull-ups
5. 5 pull-ups
6. 5 pull-ups
7. 4 pull-ups
8. 4 pull-ups
9. 4 pull-ups
10. 3 fundamental pull-ups with a 10 second descend.

If you completed this workout, head to Gorilla Group Workout 6 for your next session. If not, stick with this one until you complete it.

Glasses of water drank today: 1-2-3-4-5-6-7-8-9-10

Hours of sleep last night: 1-2-3-4-5-6-7-8-9-10

Diet: junk food————semi-healthy————healthy

Gorilla Group Workout 6

Welcome to the Gorilla Group Workout 6.

For this workout, you have 10 sets with 90 seconds of rest between each set.

Remember to focus on proper form throughout your sets.

Sets:

1. 5 pull-ups
2. 6 pull-ups
3. 5 pull-ups
4. 5 pull-ups
5. 5 pull-ups
6. 5 pull-ups
7. 5 pull-ups
8. 5 pull-ups
9. 5 pull-ups
10. Max out: perform as many pull-ups as you can.

Max reps: _____

Since this is the end of a two-week period, it is time to redo your pull-up assessment to check your progress if you fully completed this workout.

Rest a day and give the assessment a go to see which Group you will be in next.

Glasses of water drank today: 1-2-3-4-5-6-7-8-9-10

Hours of sleep last night: 1-2-3-4-5-6-7-8-9-10

Diet: junk food—————semi-healthy—————healthy

Viking Group Workouts

Viking Group Workout 1

Welcome to the Viking Group Workout 1.

For this workout, you have 6 sets with 120 seconds of rest between each set.

Remember to focus on proper form throughout your sets.

Sets:

1. 8 pull-ups
2. 8 pull-ups
3. 8 pull-ups
4. 8 pull-ups
5. 8 pull-ups
6. 2 fundamental pull-ups with a 10 second descend.

If you completed this workout, head to Viking Group Workout 2 for your next session. If not, stick with this one until you complete it.

Glasses of water drank today: 1-2-3-4-5-6-7-8-9-10

Hours of sleep last night: 1-2-3-4-5-6-7-8-9-10

Diet: junk food————semi-healthy————healthy

Viking Group Workout 2

Welcome to the Viking Group Workout 2.

For this workout, you have 9 sets with 90 seconds of rest between each set.

Remember to focus on proper form throughout your sets.

Sets:

1. 5 pull-ups
2. 6 pull-ups
3. 6 pull-ups
4. 6 pull-ups
5. 5 pull-ups
6. 5 pull-ups
7. 5 pull-ups
8. 5 pull-ups
9. 3 fundamental pull-ups with a 10 second descend.

If you completed this workout, head to Viking Group Workout 3 for your next session. If not, stick with this one until you complete it.

Glasses of water drank today: 1-2-3-4-5-6-7-8-9-10

Hours of sleep last night: 1-2-3-4-5-6-7-8-9-10

Diet: junk food————semi-healthy————healthy

Viking Group Workout 3

Welcome to the Viking Group Workout 3.

For this workout, you have 9 sets with 90 seconds of rest between each set.

Remember to focus on proper form throughout your sets.

Sets:

1. 6 pull-ups
2. 7 pull-ups
3. 7 pull-ups
4. 7 pull-ups
5. 6 pull-ups
6. 6 pull-ups
7. 6 pull-ups
8. 6 pull-ups
9. Max out: perform as many pull-ups as you can.

Max reps: _____

If you completed this workout, head to Viking Group Workout 4 for your next session. If not, stick with this one until you complete it.

Glasses of water drank today: 1-2-3-4-5-6-7-8-9-10

Hours of sleep last night: 1-2-3-4-5-6-7-8-9-10

Diet: junk food—————semi-healthy—————healthy

Viking Group Workout 4

Welcome to the Viking Group Workout 4.

For this workout, you have 6 sets with 120 seconds of rest between each set.

Remember to focus on proper form throughout your sets.

Sets:

1. 11 pull-ups
2. 11 pull-ups
3. 11 pull-ups
4. 11 pull-ups
5. 11 pull-ups
6. 3 fundamental pull-ups with a 10 second descend.

If you completed this workout, head to Viking Group Workout 5 for your next session. If not, stick with this one until you complete it.

Glasses of water drank today: 1-2-3-4-5-6-7-8-9-10

Hours of sleep last night: 1-2-3-4-5-6-7-8-9-10

Diet: junk food————semi-healthy————healthy

Viking Group Workout 5

Welcome to the Viking Group Workout 5.

For this workout, you have 10 sets with 90 seconds of rest between each set.

Remember to focus on proper form throughout your sets.

Sets:

1. 6 pull-ups
2. 7 pull-ups
3. 7 pull-ups
4. 7 pull-ups
5. 7 pull-ups
6. 7 pull-ups
7. 6 pull-ups
8. 6 pull-ups
9. 6 pull-ups
10. 4 fundamental pull-ups with a 10 second descend.

If you completed this workout, head to Viking Group Workout 6 for your next session. If not, stick with this one until you complete it.

Glasses of water drank today: 1-2-3-4-5-6-7-8-9-10

Hours of sleep last night: 1-2-3-4-5-6-7-8-9-10

Diet: junk food—————semi-healthy—————healthy

Viking Group Workout 6

Welcome to the Viking Group Workout 6.

For this workout, you have 10 sets with 90 seconds of rest between each set.

Remember to focus on proper form throughout your sets.

Sets:

1. 7 pull-ups
2. 8 pull-ups
3. 8 pull-ups
4. 8 pull-ups
5. 7 pull-ups
6. 7 pull-ups
7. 7 pull-ups
8. 7 pull-ups
9. 7 pull-ups
10. Max out: perform as many pull-ups as you can.

Max reps: _____

Since this is the end of a two-week period, it is time to redo your pull-up assessment to check your progress if you fully completed this workout.

Rest a day and give the assessment a go to see which Group you will be in next.

Glasses of water drank today: 1-2-3-4-5-6-7-8-9-10

Hours of sleep last night: 1-2-3-4-5-6-7-8-9-10

Diet: junk food————semi-healthy————healthy

Elite Group Workouts

Elite Group Workout 1

Welcome to the Elite Group Workout 1.

For this workout, you have 6 sets with 120 seconds of rest between each set.

Remember to focus on proper form throughout your sets.

Sets:

1. 10 pull-ups
2. 10 pull-ups
3. 10 pull-ups
4. 10 pull-ups
5. 10 pull-ups
6. 3 fundamental pull-ups with a 10 second descend.

If you completed this workout, head to Elite Group Workout 2 for your next session. If not, stick with this one until you complete it.

Glasses of water drank today: 1-2-3-4-5-6-7-8-9-10

Hours of sleep last night: 1-2-3-4-5-6-7-8-9-10

Diet: junk food—————semi-healthy—————healthy

Elite Group Workout 2

Welcome to the Elite Group Workout 2.

For this workout, you have 9 sets with 90 seconds of rest between each set.

Remember to focus on proper form throughout your sets.

Sets:

1. 6 pull-ups
2. 7 pull-ups
3. 7 pull-ups
4. 7 pull-ups
5. 6 pull-ups
6. 6 pull-ups
7. 6 pull-ups
8. 6 pull-ups
9. 3 fundamental pull-ups with a 10 second descend.

If you completed this workout, head to Elite Group Workout 3 for your next session. If not, stick with this one until you complete it.

Glasses of water drank today: 1-2-3-4-5-6-7-8-9-10

Hours of sleep last night: 1-2-3-4-5-6-7-8-9-10

Diet: junk food————semi-healthy————healthy

Elite Group Workout 3

Welcome to the Elite Group Workout 3.

For this workout, you have 9 sets with 90 seconds of rest between each set.

Remember to focus on proper form throughout your sets.

Sets:

1. 7 pull-ups
2. 8 pull-ups
3. 8 pull-ups
4. 8 pull-ups
5. 7 pull-ups
6. 7 pull-ups
7. 7 pull-ups
8. 7 pull-ups
9. Max out: perform as many pull-ups as you can.

Max reps: _____

If you completed this workout, head to Elite Group Workout 4 for your next session. If not, stick with this one until you complete it.

Glasses of water drank today: 1-2-3-4-5-6-7-8-9-10

Hours of sleep last night: 1-2-3-4-5-6-7-8-9-10

Diet: junk food—————semi-healthy—————healthy

Elite Group Workout 4

Welcome to the Elite Group Workout 4.

For this workout, you have 6 sets with 120 seconds of rest between each set.

Remember to focus on proper form throughout your sets.

Sets:

1. 12 pull-ups
2. 12 pull-ups
3. 12 pull-ups
4. 12 pull-ups
5. 12 pull-ups
6. 4 fundamental pull-ups with a 10 second descend.

If you completed this workout, head to Elite Group Workout 5 for your next session. If not, stick with this one until you complete it.

Glasses of water drank today: 1-2-3-4-5-6-7-8-9-10

Hours of sleep last night: 1-2-3-4-5-6-7-8-9-10

Diet: junk food————semi-healthy————healthy

Elite Group Workout 5

Welcome to the Elite Group Workout 5.

For this workout, you have 10 sets with 90 seconds of rest between each set.

Remember to focus on proper form throughout your sets.

Sets:

1. 7 pull-ups
2. 8 pull-ups
3. 8 pull-ups
4. 8 pull-ups
5. 8 pull-ups
6. 8 pull-ups
7. 7 pull-ups
8. 7 pull-ups
9. 7 pull-ups
10. 4 fundamental pull-ups with a 10 second descend.

If you completed this workout, head to Elite Group Workout 6 for your next session. If not, stick with this one until you complete it.

Glasses of water drank today: 1-2-3-4-5-6-7-8-9-10

Hours of sleep last night: 1-2-3-4-5-6-7-8-9-10

Diet: junk food————semi-healthy————healthy

Elite Group Workout 6

Welcome to the Elite Group Workout 6.

For this workout, you have 10 sets with 90 seconds of rest between each set.

[Remember to focus on proper form throughout your sets.

Sets:

1. 8 pull-ups
2. 9 pull-ups
3. 9 pull-ups
4. 9 pull-ups
5. 8 pull-ups
6. 8 pull-ups
7. 8 pull-ups
8. 8 pull-ups
9. 8 pull-ups
10. Max out: perform as many pull-ups as you can.

Max reps: _____

Since this is the end of a two-week period, it is time to redo your pull-up assessment to check your progress if you fully completed this workout.

Rest a day and give the assessment a go to see which Group you will be in next.

Glasses of water drank today: 1-2-3-4-5-6-7-8-9-10

Hours of sleep last night: 1-2-3-4-5-6-7-8-9-10

Diet: junk food———––semi-healthy———––healthy

Commando Group Workouts

Commando Group Workout 1

Welcome to the Commando Group Workout 1.

For this workout, you have 6 sets with 120 seconds of rest between each set.

Remember to focus on proper form throughout your sets.

Sets:

1. 9 pull-ups
2. 9 pull-ups
3. 9 pull-ups
4. 9 pull-ups
5. 9 pull-ups
6. 4 fundamental pull-ups with a 10 second descend.

If you completed this workout, head to Commando Group Workout 2 for your next session. If not, stick with this one until you complete it.

Glasses of water drank today: 1-2-3-4-5-6-7-8-9-10

Hours of sleep last night: 1-2-3-4-5-6-7-8-9-10

Diet: junk food————semi-healthy————healthy

Commando Group Workout 2

Welcome to the Commando Group Workout 2.

For this workout, you have 10 sets with 90 seconds of rest between each set.

Remember to focus on proper form throughout your sets.

Sets:

1. 5 pull-ups
2. 6 pull-ups
3. 6 pull-ups
4. 6 pull-ups
5. 5 pull-ups
6. 5 pull-ups
7. 5 pull-ups
8. 5 pull-ups
9. 5 pull-ups
10. 4 fundamental pull-ups with a 10 second descend.

If you completed this workout, head to Commando Group Workout 3 for your next session. If not, stick with this one until you complete it.

Glasses of water drank today: 1-2-3-4-5-6-7-8-9-10

Hours of sleep last night: 1-2-3-4-5-6-7-8-9-10

Diet: junk food————semi-healthy————healthy

Commando Group Workout 3

Welcome to the Commando Group Workout 3.

For this workout, you have 10 sets with 90 seconds of rest between each set.

Remember to focus on proper form throughout your sets.

Sets:

1. 5 pull-ups
2. 6 pull-ups
3. 6 pull-ups
4. 6 pull-ups
5. 6 pull-ups
6. 6 pull-ups
7. 5 pull-ups
8. 5 pull-ups
9. 5 pull-ups
10. Max out: perform as many pull-ups as you can.

Max reps: _____

If you completed this workout, head to Commando Group Workout 4 for your next session. If not, stick with this one until you complete it.

Glasses of water drank today: 1-2-3-4-5-6-7-8-9-10

Hours of sleep last night: 1-2-3-4-5-6-7-8-9-10

Diet: junk food————semi-healthy————healthy

Commando Group Workout 4

Welcome to the Commando Group Workout 4.

For this workout, you have 6 sets with 120 seconds of rest between each set.

Remember to focus on proper form throughout your sets.

Sets:

1. 12 pull-ups
2. 12 pull-ups
3. 12 pull-ups
4. 12 pull-ups
5. 12 pull-ups
6. 5 fundamental pull-ups with a 10 second descend.

If you completed this workout, head to Commando Group Workout 5 for your next session. If not, stick with this one until you complete it.

Glasses of water drank today: 1-2-3-4-5-6-7-8-9-10

Hours of sleep last night: 1-2-3-4-5-6-7-8-9-10

Diet: junk food—————semi-healthy—————healthy

Commando Group Workout 5

Welcome to the Commando Group Workout 5.

For this workout, you have 10 sets with 90 seconds of rest between each set.

Remember to focus on proper form throughout your sets.

Sets:

1. 6 pull-ups
2. 7 pull-ups
3. 7 pull-ups
4. 7 pull-ups
5. 6 pull-ups
6. 6 pull-ups
7. 6 pull-ups
8. 6 pull-ups
9. 6 pull-ups
10. 5 fundamental pull-ups with a 10 second descend.

If you completed this workout, head to Commando Group Workout 6 for your next session. If not, stick with this one until you complete it.

Glasses of water drank today: 1-2-3-4-5-6-7-8-9-10

Hours of sleep last night: 1-2-3-4-5-6-7-8-9-10

Diet: junk food—————semi-healthy—————healthy

Commando Group Workout 6

Welcome to the Commando Group Workout 6.

For this workout, you have 10 sets with 90 seconds of rest between each set.

Remember to focus on proper form throughout your sets.

Sets:

1. 6 pull-ups
2. 7 pull-ups
3. 7 pull-ups
4. 7 pull-ups
5. 6 pull-ups
6. 6 pull-ups
7. 6 pull-ups
8. 6 pull-ups
9. 6 pull-ups
10. Max out: perform as many pull-ups as you can.

Max reps: _____

If you completed this workout, you have earned the right to attempt 30 consecutive pull-ups. Take a few days off to fully recover and take a shot at hitting your goal.

You got this.

Glasses of water drank today: 1-2-3-4-5-6-7-8-9-10

Hours of sleep last night: 1-2-3-4-5-6-7-8-9-10

Diet: junk food————semi-healthy————healthy

Veteran Group Workouts

Veteran Group Workout 1

Welcome to the Veteran Group Workout 1.

For this workout, you have 6 sets with 120 seconds of rest between each set.

Remember to focus on proper form throughout your sets.

Sets:

1. 13 pull-ups
2. 13 pull-ups
3. 13 pull-ups
4. 13 pull-ups
5. 13 pull-ups
6. 4 fundamental pull-ups with a 10 second descend.

If you completed this workout, head to Veteran Group Workout 2 for your next session. If not, stick with this one until you complete it.

Glasses of water drank today: 1-2-3-4-5-6-7-8-9-10

Hours of sleep last night: 1-2-3-4-5-6-7-8-9-10

Diet: junk food————semi-healthy————healthy

Veteran Group Workout 2

Welcome to the Veteran Group Workout 2.

For this workout, you have 10 sets with 90 seconds of rest between each set.

Remember to focus on proper form throughout your sets.

Sets:

1. 7 pull-ups
2. 8 pull-ups
3. 8 pull-ups
4. 8 pull-ups
5. 8 pull-ups
6. 8 pull-ups
7. 7 pull-ups
8. 7 pull-ups
9. 7 pull-ups
10. 4 fundamental pull-ups with a 10 second descend.

If you completed this workout, head to Veteran Group Workout 3 for your next session. If not, stick with this one until you complete it.

Glasses of water drank today: 1-2-3-4-5-6-7-8-9-10

Hours of sleep last night: 1-2-3-4-5-6-7-8-9-10

Diet: junk food————semi-healthy————healthy

Veteran Group Workout 3

Welcome to the Veteran Group Workout 3.

For this workout, you have 10 sets with 90 seconds of rest between each set.

Remember to focus on proper form throughout your sets.

Sets:

1. 8 pull-ups
2. 9 pull-ups
3. 9 pull-ups
4. 9 pull-ups
5. 8 pull-ups
6. 8 pull-ups
7. 8 pull-ups
8. 8 pull-ups
9. 8 pull-ups
10. Max out: perform as many pull-ups as you can.

Max reps: _____

If you completed this workout, head to Veteran Group Workout 4 for your next session. If not, stick with this one until you complete it.

Glasses of water drank today: 1-2-3-4-5-6-7-8-9-10

Hours of sleep last night: 1-2-3-4-5-6-7-8-9-10

Diet: junk food————semi-healthy————healthy

Veteran Group Workout 4

Welcome to the Veteran Group Workout 4.

For this workout, you have 6 sets with 120 seconds of rest between each set.

Remember to focus on proper form throughout your sets.

Sets:

1. 16 pull-ups
2. 16 pull-ups
3. 16 pull-ups
4. 16 pull-ups
5. 16 pull-ups
6. 5 fundamental pull-ups with a 10 second descend.

If you completed this workout, head to Veteran Group Workout 5 for your next session. If not, stick with this one until you complete it.

Glasses of water drank today: 1-2-3-4-5-6-7-8-9-10

Hours of sleep last night: 1-2-3-4-5-6-7-8-9-10

Diet: junk food————semi-healthy————healthy

Veteran Group Workout 5

Welcome to the Veteran Group Workout 5.

For this workout, you have 10 sets with 90 seconds of rest between each set.

Remember to focus on proper form throughout your sets.

Sets:

1. 8 pull-ups
2. 9 pull-ups
3. 9 pull-ups
4. 9 pull-ups
5. 9 pull-ups
6. 9 pull-ups
7. 8 pull-ups
8. 8 pull-ups
9. 8 pull-ups
10. 5 fundamental pull-ups with a 10 second descend.

If you completed this workout, head to Veteran Group Workout 6 for your next session. If not, stick with this one until you complete it.

Glasses of water drank today: 1-2-3-4-5-6-7-8-9-10

Hours of sleep last night: 1-2-3-4-5-6-7-8-9-10

Diet: junk food—————semi-healthy—————healthy

Veteran Group Workout 6

Welcome to the Veteran Group Workout 6.

For this workout, you have 10 sets with 90 seconds of rest between each set.

Remember to focus on proper form throughout your sets.

Sets:

1. 9 pull-ups
2. 10 pull-ups
3. 10 pull-ups
4. 10 pull-ups
5. 9 pull-ups
6. 9 pull-ups
7. 9 pull-ups
8. 9 pull-ups
9. 9 pull-ups
10. Max out: perform as many pull-ups as you can.

Max reps: _____

If you completed this workout, you have earned the right to attempt 30 consecutive pull-ups. Take a few days off to fully recover and take a shot at hitting your goal.

You got this.

Glasses of water drank today: 1-2-3-4-5-6-7-8-9-10

Hours of sleep last night: 1-2-3-4-5-6-7-8-9-10

Diet: junk food—————semi-healthy—————healthy

Nuclear Group Workouts

Nuclear Group Workout 1

Welcome to the Nuclear Group Workout 1.

For this workout, you have 6 sets with 120 seconds of rest between each set.

Remember to focus on proper form throughout your sets.

Sets:

1. 15 pull-ups
2. 15 pull-ups
3. 15 pull-ups
4. 15 pull-ups
5. 15 pull-ups
6. 5 fundamental pull-ups with a 10 second descend.

If you completed this workout, head to Nuclear Group Workout 2 for your next session. If not, stick with this one until you complete it.

Glasses of water drank today: 1-2-3-4-5-6-7-8-9-10

Hours of sleep last night: 1-2-3-4-5-6-7-8-9-10

Diet: junk food—————semi-healthy—————healthy

Nuclear Group Workout 2

Welcome to the Nuclear Group Workout 2.

For this workout, you have 10 sets with 90 seconds of rest between each set.

Remember to focus on proper form throughout your sets.

Sets:

1. 8 pull-ups
2. 9 pull-ups
3. 9 pull-ups
4. 9 pull-ups
5. 9 pull-ups
6. 9 pull-ups
7. 8 pull-ups
8. 8 pull-ups
9. 8 pull-ups
10. 5 fundamental pull-ups with a 10 second descend.

If you completed this workout, head to Nuclear Group Workout 3 for your next session. If not, stick with this one until you complete it.

Glasses of water drank today: 1-2-3-4-5-6-7-8-9-10

Hours of sleep last night: 1-2-3-4-5-6-7-8-9-10

Diet: junk food—————semi-healthy—————healthy

Nuclear Group Workout 3

Welcome to the Nuclear Group Workout 3.

For this workout, you have 10 sets with 90 seconds of rest between each set.

Remember to focus on proper form throughout your sets.

Sets:

1. 9 pull-ups
2. 10 pull-ups
3. 10 pull-ups
4. 10 pull-ups
5. 9 pull-ups
6. 9 pull-ups
7. 9 pull-ups
8. 9 pull-ups
9. 9 pull-ups
10. Max out: perform as many pull-ups as you can.

Max reps: _____

If you completed this workout, head to Nuclear Group Workout 4 for your next session. If not, stick with this one until you complete it.

Glasses of water drank today: 1-2-3-4-5-6-7-8-9-10

Hours of sleep last night: 1-2-3-4-5-6-7-8-9-10

Diet: junk food————semi-healthy————healthy

Nuclear Group Workout 4

Welcome to the Nuclear Group Workout 4.

For this workout, you have 6 sets with 120 seconds of rest between each set.

Remember to focus on proper form throughout your sets.

Sets:

1. 18 pull-ups
2. 18 pull-ups
3. 18 pull-ups
4. 18 pull-ups
5. 18 pull-ups
6. 5 fundamental pull-ups with a 10 second descend.

If you completed this workout, head to Nuclear Group Workout 5 for your next session. If not, stick with this one until you complete it.

Glasses of water drank today: 1-2-3-4-5-6-7-8-9-10

Hours of sleep last night: 1-2-3-4-5-6-7-8-9-10

Diet: junk food————semi-healthy————healthy

Nuclear Group Workout 5

Welcome to the Nuclear Group Workout 5.

For this workout, you have 10 sets with 90 seconds of rest between each set.

Remember to focus on proper form throughout your sets.

Sets:

1. 9 pull-ups
2. 10 pull-ups
3. 10 pull-ups
4. 10 pull-ups
5. 10 pull-ups
6. 10 pull-ups
7. 9 pull-ups
8. 9 pull-ups
9. 9 pull-ups
10. 5 fundamental pull-ups with a 10 second descend.

If you completed this workout, head to Nuclear Group Workout 6 for your next session. If not, stick with this one until you complete it.

Glasses of water drank today: 1-2-3-4-5-6-7-8-9-10

Hours of sleep last night: 1-2-3-4-5-6-7-8-9-10

Diet: junk food—————semi-healthy—————healthy

Nuclear Group Workout 6

Welcome to the Nuclear Group Workout 6.

For this workout, you have 10 sets with 90 seconds of rest between each set.

Remember to focus on proper form throughout your sets.

Sets:

1. 10 pull-ups
2. 11 pull-ups
3. 11 pull-ups
4. 11 pull-ups
5. 11 pull-ups
6. 11 pull-ups
7. 10 pull-ups
8. 10 pull-ups
9. 10 pull-ups
10. Max out: perform as many pull-ups as you can.

Max reps: _____

If you completed this workout, you have earned the right to attempt 30 consecutive pull-ups. Take a few days off to fully recover and take a shot at hitting your goal.

You got this.

Glasses of water drank today: 1-2-3-4-5-6-7-8-9-10

Hours of sleep last night: 1-2-3-4-5-6-7-8-9-10

Diet: junk food———––semi-healthy———––healthy

Attempting 30 Consecutive Pull-ups

If you are here, that means you have completed either the Commando, Veteran, or Nuclear Group Workouts and have earned the right to attempt 30 consecutive pull-ups.

Your goal is well within your grasp and all you have to do is take it.

As you begin to warm up to crush this, I'd like to ask a favor.

I'm going to be greedy for a minute here and ask you to leave a review for the book.

Reviews are a pain to get but it will only take a minute or two to leave one.

Scan this QR which will take you straight to the book's page on Amazon.

Scroll down and click the 'leave a customer review' button, select your star rating, leave a few words, and that is it!

It is that simple!

Once that is done, get ready to crush this.

Get psyched for what is about to happen.

Give it everything you have got to knock out as many correct pull-ups without stopping.

Once you are done, come back.

* * *

If you nailed 30 or more, awesome.

That is incredible. Time to knock that off your bucket list.

If you didn't quite get it, no worries. Not everyone gets it on the first try.

Use this number as your new assessment number and get back at it!

Cheers.

Conclusion:

I just want to thank you for making your way through this program and the book. You have bettered yourself for it.

I hope you have challenged yourself and I hope you tasted victory by reaching 30 consecutive pull-ups.

If you are hungry for more challenges, we've got plenty more where this came from.

And if you have enjoyed this book, do take a second to leave a review.

Until next time.

Cheers.